Published By Adam Gilbin

@ Corey Kidd

Chakras: Energy Healing, and Creating a Balanced

Life Empowering Prayers and Affi Rmations for

Balance

All Right RESERVED

ISBN 978-87-94477-73-4

TABLE OF CONTENTS

Chapter 1 1

The History Of Chakras: Tracing The Origins And Development Over Time 1

Chapter 2 5

Understanding The Basics 5

Chapter 3 Sacral Chakra - Creativity 16

Chapter 4 23

Clearing Your Mind To Enhance Your Creativity 23

Chapter 5 32

The Crown Chakra: Your Cosmic Portal 32

Chapter 6 43

Muladhara 43

Chapter 7 47

Open Your Root Chakra With Yoga 47

Chapter 8 57

Chakras' Teachings: 57

A Path To Life Transformation. 57

Chapter 9 77

Some Of The Life Lessons Of The Seven Major Chakras: 77

Chapter 10 84

The Primary Seven Chakras 84

Chapter 11 90

What Is Muladhara? 90

Chapter 12 110

Identify Your Imbalance 110

Chapter 13 130

Finding Your Imbalance Via Meditation 130

Chapter 14 Throat Chakra - Communication 138

CHAPTER 1

The History of Chakras: Tracing the Origins and Development Over Time

In our pursuit of understanding chakras and their significance in the modern world, it is imperative to start on a journey into their historical and cultural origins. The history of chakras is a tapestry woven with ancient wisdom, spirituality, and cultural influences, and it is within this tapestry that we can uncover the timeless nature of these mystical energy centers.

Ancient Roots of Chakras:

Our exploration begins in the heart of ancient India, where the earliest known references to chakras can be found. These references date back to the Vedic period, between 1500 and 500 BCE, in sacred texts known as the Vedas. In these early writings, chakras were described as fundamental centers of energy and consciousness, deeply interconnected with the human body, mind, and spirit.

Development in Hinduism and Tantra:

As we trace the historical evolution of chakras, we find that their significance grew within the context of Hinduism and Tantra. Chakras became integral components of the subtle body, featuring prominently in yoga and meditation practices. Each chakra was associated with specific qualities, elements, and even divine deities. This development added layers of complexity to the understanding and use of chakras in spiritual and mystical contexts.

Spread to Other Cultures:

Chakras did not remain confined to the boundaries of India. Over time, this concept found its way into other cultures and spiritual traditions. Tibetan Buddhism, in particular, embraced chakras as part of the Vajrayana path, where they became central to practices like Tummo meditation. Similarly, Chinese Qigong and Japanese Reiki incorporated chakra-like energy centres into their own systems, highlighting the universal appeal and adaptability of chakra concepts.

The Western Encounter:
The history of chakras took an intriguing turn in the Western world during the late 19th and early 20th centuries. Influenced by Theosophy, a spiritual and philosophical movement, and figures like Helena Blavatsky and C.W. Leadbeater, Western audiences were introduced to the concept of chakras. These writings played a

significant role in popularizing chakras and influenced the development of Western energy healing practices, setting the stage for the New Age movements that emerged in the 20th century.

Contemporary Relevance:

Today, the history of chakras has brought us to a point where these energy centers continue to be of immense relevance in our lives. Chakras have undergone a process of fusion, where Eastern and Western perspectives have merged to shape contemporary understanding. They are now embraced in various practices, from yoga and meditation to energy healing, holistic wellness, and personal development.

CHAPTER 2

Understanding The Basics

The next day, in her dreams, the sage praised her for her consistency. And was also amazed to see a paper and pencil in her hand. Arya was enthusiastic and ready to take notes on all the things she had to learn. Sage laughed and said, you know why I am there in your dreams and have not encountered you in real life? She looked perplexed, clearly suggesting no. The sage continued; it is because every answer you seek lies within you. When you meditate, you get all the answers from within. Arya had a blissful experience just listening to these words. She felt a sense of empowerment and curiosity as she realized that she held the key to unlocking her own wisdom. Intrigued by the sage's words, she made a silent promise to herself to explore meditation and discover the answers that resided within her own being.

Arya began to ask, I am ready to grasp the concept; please make me understand it, as she was curious to learn more about the idea of chakra balancing. The sage smiled warmly at her eagerness and began to explain:

According to the yogic scriptures, we have two bodies within us: the physical body and the spiritual body. Our physical body is what we see; it ends at our skin and hairs, but the spiritual body extends 2–5 cm around our physical body. That's how we have an aura around us. Some people have a more radiating and well-defined aura; those are spiritually awakened beings. And the rest of us have less well-defined auras. These two bodies largely overlap. Therefore, we will refer to them collectively as our bodies. Our bodies, both physical and spiritual, are interconnected and influence each other in various ways. While our physical body is tangible and visible, our spiritual body encompasses our emotions, thoughts, and energy. Understanding the existence of these two bodies allows us to explore deeper aspects of ourselves and the world around us.

Arya astonishingly questioned, everyone around us knows the physical body basics pretty well: the eyes, nose, hands, etc. What is our spiritual body composed of? The Sage replied, our spiritual body has 114 energy centers within it, and among those seven are prominent ones. Just like our physical body has organs to interact with the outer world, these seven energy centers are the sense organs of our soul. And by stimulating them, we can live a more soulful life. Just as a person goes to the gym or practices yoga to keep the muscles flexed, we need to stimulate these chakras to keep the soul enlightened.

Arya listened intently, her curiosity growing with each word, eager to embark on this new journey of self-discovery. The Sage continued: These 7 energy sense organs are the 7 chakras inside you; you can think of chakras as the places in your body where energy is concentrated. These seven chakras have seven different kinds of energies concentrated in them. They are like batteries that store and distribute energy throughout your system. They are aligned along your spine from the tail bone to the crown of your head. Each chakra has a location and a function.

The first chakra is the root chakra **(Muladhar)**. It is located at the bottom of your tailbone. It governs your productivity, your survival instincts, your physical security, and your connection to nature. The second chakra is the sacral chakra (**Svadhisthan**). It is located just below your navel, in your lower abdomen. It governs your emotions, your creativity, and your sexuality. The third chakra is called the solar plexus chakra . It is located in your upper abdomen, between your navel and your sternum. It governs your willpower, your confidence, and your personal power. The gut feeling is also associated with this chakra. The fourth chakra is called the heart chakra **(Anahat)**. It is located in the center of your chest, near your heart. It governs your love, your compassion, and your joy. The fifth chakra is called the throat chakra **(Vishuddh)**. It is located in your throat area. It governs your communication, your expression, your truth, and your ability to forgive. The sixth chakra is called the third eye chakra **(Ajna).** It is located in the center of your forehead, in between your eyebrows. It governs your intuition, your vision, your wisdom, and your intellect. The seventh chakra is called the crown chakra **(Sahasrar)**. It is located in the center, right above your head. Remember that your spiritual body extends beyond your physical body. It governs your spirituality, your connection to the divine, to the universe, and to yourself.

After the information flow, the sage paused for any questions that Arya had. As curious as she was, she was also a bit nervous about delving into such deep spiritual concepts. However, her curiosity got the better of her, and she mustered up the courage to ask a question.

Arya: You told me so much about the 7 chakras and didn't allow me to take notes; how am I supposed to remember all this? Just as a child, you find it challenging to learn and retain anything, Sage remarked lightheartedly. Consider memorizing body parts and failing to remember them all throughout tests. And you now recall each one when someone asks you about it. You get used to learning. Similar to this, if you begin to practice chakra balancing, you'll get used to it, and the information will stick with you naturally.

Arya: You also mentioned the interconnection of the spiritual body with the physical body, but you only shared the intangible aspects related to each chakra. The sage responded, You missed the point where I mentioned the location of each chakra with respect to the physical body. Non the less, let me also make you aware of the organs and glands that are directly affected by each chakra. Whenever you face issues with any of the organs or glands, try balancing the corresponding chakra. You will see incredible results.

Root chakra: This chakra is located at the base of the spine and is associated with the testes, kidneys, spine, and adrenal glands.

Sacral chakra: This chakra is located below the navel and is associated with the bladder, prostate, ovaries, kidneys, gall bladder, bowel, spleen, and reproductive organs.

Solar plexus chakra: This chakra is located above the navel and is associated with the pancreas, stomach, liver, spleen, and digestive system.

Heart chakra: This chakra is located in the center of the chest and is associated with the thymus gland, heart, lungs, and circulatory system.

Throat chakra: This chakra is located at the base of the throat and is associated with the thyroid gland, vocal cords, mouth, ears, and respiratory system.

Third eye chakra: This chakra is located between the eyebrows and is associated with the pituitary gland, hypothalamus, eyes, and brain.

Crown chakra: This chakra is located at the top of the head and is associated with the pineal gland, nervous system, and cerebral cortex.

Arya: So this is how we treat bodily ailments?

Sage: Generally speaking, yes. I make this statement because physical ailments require physical treatment for their physical symptoms. Chakra balancing techniques will aid in recuperation, speed up healing by a large amount, and in mild situations of organ dysfunction, they can completely restore health.

Arya: Sounds reasonable. Although I am aware of the need for balance in our lives, you are constantly referring to balancing routines. But I've also heard of things like chakra opening and awakening. Sage: According to popular belief, a chakra's ability to receive or transmit energy and how well it functions determine whether it is open or closed. This is a simplification nonetheless and does not reflect the dynamic and complex nature of the chakras. According to Arhanta Yoga, chakras are always active and in motion, but they can be balanced or imbalanced, overactive or underactive, harmonious or disharmonious. The goal of chakra balancing is not open or close the chakras but to bring them into alignment and harmony with each other and with the universal energy.

Arya: And what about the balancing routines and seven chakras you explained? Do they fall out of balance at once? Sage: No, the chakras can fall out of balance individually or in combination with each other. It is common for one or more chakras to be imbalanced while the others remain in harmony. The balancing routines aim to identify and address these imbalances to restore overall energetic equilibrium. How about you coming tomorrow again so we can take our lessons one step further to identify the imbalances? Arya: That sounds like a great idea! I'm excited to continue our lessons and delve deeper into identifying and addressing the imbalances in my chakras. I believe it will help me achieve a greater sense of energetic harmony and well-being.

Chapter 3

Sacral Chakra - Creativity

I am learning that the power of expressing myself can only be found if I am willing to break free from my comfort zone and into a space that allows me to be completely liberated. I am ready to fully embrace this freedom.

This chapter describes what the sacral chakra is, how it can be activated, and how you can use your energy to express your creativity. As many people find it harder by the day to keep up with most of their interests, a blockage has suffered in the sacral chakra. A lack of creating ideas to bring to life sinks some people into a state of dullness, where they may begin to stop expressing themselves even in other aspects of their lives. Some of the questions that this chapter will attempt to address include:

- What is the sacral chakra?

- What is creativity?
- How do you meditate to clear your mind?
- How can you enhance and move your creative energy techniques through the sacral chakra?

What Is the Sacral Chakra?

The sacral chakra is closest to your navel, where it is responsible for your happiness, reproductive system, passion, and the enhancement of your creativity through multiple forms of expression. Fear can cause a blockage of this chakra, as it interrupts the flow emphasized by this chakra. The sacral chakra is also known as the Swadhisthana (where the self dwells), and water is the element that is linked to this chakra. Your sacral chakra encourages you to realize your potential by exploring as much as you possibly can. It is similar to your inner child, where it is constantly seeking to do whatever sets your spirit free. Orange is the color associated with this chakra, along with the 417 Hz solfeggio frequency that helps eliminate blockages and accept change in your life. Traumatic experiences you might have experienced in the past may start to clear up when you use the 417 Hz frequency or the note 'Re' since the effects you might still feel will gradually diminish. This frequency will enable a shift of energy in the sacral chakra that will assist in a shift of your mental state. Feelings such as frustration or dissatisfaction that you might confine yourself to will require that you liberate yourself mentally from any unnecessary bondages.

If you are fond of nature, you may want to go to places that have waterfalls, fountains, streams, or rivers to heighten the power of the sacral chakra. The calming effect that water bodies have serves as a reminder of the harmony that flows throughout our bodies, which comprise approximately 60% of water. When sitting outdoors, try to listen to as many sounds in your surroundings as possible so that once you are in complete silence, you can activate your mental 'tape recorder' to replay all of those sounds. Connections to the sounds in our surroundings, especially in their most natural states, such as hearing the sound of chirping birds, a hooter of a car going off, a plane flying above your head in the sky, or the sound of air flowing about can help you increase your alertness. The sensations that may arise from these sounds could also help you understand parts of yourself that respond to these sounds.

You will be allowed to learn just how much responsibility you have over your responses or reactions to, through, and with yourself, and whatever surroundings you may be immersed in at that moment. Try to sit across the sun just before 5 p.m. to observe any feelings or thoughts that pace through your mind. Sit as comfortably as you can on the ground. The feelings or thoughts you have during this moment of connecting with yourself will vary, so you should not focus only on one feeling or thought but try to have a collective experience of them all. You will notice how sitting in complete silence can gradually become something you practice daily, even with other surrounding noises. These external interferences may start to get blocked out by your consciousness rising. You may also experience moments throughout your day when these moments with yourself become somewhat of a feeling or thought that you could return to without needing to physically be there.

Another method of activating your sacral chakra is by giving yourself sensual massages along your body. These may also activate your sensual energy and alert your mind to your awareness. The need for changing how you open yourself up to receiving these sensations from your partner could also be stimulated in the same way. There may be a tingling of sexual energy when you move the energy up from your stomach to your third eye, as you will feel this energy at the center of your forehead. Your ability to raise your awareness is dependent on your willingness to carry this energy throughout your whole body.

While intimacy is desirable for people of age, the more you are sexually active, the more your mental power may diminish. This is why it is important to direct your sexual energy needs toward a release for blocked-up energy rather than a fulfillment of lust or underlying depression. In addition, people who experience hypersexuality may, more often than not, be experiencing unprocessed sexual trauma, a need for acceptance or recognition, and sexual intercourse could be how they suppress feelings that need to be addressed accordingly. This should not, however, discourage you from unleashing your sexual energy since this is simply guidance on how releasing your sexual energy should be carried out in moderation.

The relationships and connections you have with yourself and others require your honesty of your experience with them. You need to start asking yourself:
Whether or not these are toxic or platonic relationships
If your friendships buckle under certain circumstances and why this may be the case
Or even why you struggle to remain in stable intimate relationships
When your sacral chakra is experiencing blockages, you will need to evaluate these situations closely so that you can eliminate the imbalance in your life and clear your mind from any clutter.

Chapter 4

Clearing Your Mind to Enhance Your Creativity

A cluttered mind has no room to breed anything new. Therefore, you cannot attempt to usher in a new wave of energy if you have not cleared all the energy that had previously blocked your chakras. New ideas and interests are developed from a fresh perspective, so you cannot transform your energy balance if you still keep to old living patterns.

To create the desired flow of energy to activate the sacral chakra, you can chant the word Vam or use the expression 'I feel...' to describe how or what you are feeling. Try to limit harboring your feelings since this will only backfire on you at the most unexpected time. When you allow yourself to feel every emotion that springs your way, you subconsciously acknowledge that it is okay to feel this way. From that point, you would have identified where the feeling came from and began finding ways to address these feelings so that they are not harbored within you. Not expressing your feelings prevents you from expressing yourself in other ways, especially through creativity. So, you might want to ensure that your sacral chakra remains unblocked. You could be surprised to learn that this can also be the starting point for welcoming change into your life, particularly through a transformed outlook on life. This is how you can gain a 'new lease on life' and begin to live a life where you are constantly meeting your true self.

An example of a technique that you can use as a daily practice is to close your eyes and imagine a blank canvas. This canvas should be viewed as your life. So, what you visually apply to the canvas is what you will ultimately apply to your life. As you start filling up your canvas, think of everything you want to see on the finished artwork. This visualization will translate into feelings, and you should pay careful attention to these. Once you feel you are done, speak life into whatever has filled your canvas, and as you slowly reopen your eyes, you might still have pieces of that canvas appearing in your waking world. This happens as it will stimulate the activation of your sacral chakra in the process, and the creative energy will still be creating a vibrational force throughout your body and mind. The memory of this canvas will remain with you as long as you keep it in your visions since you would have created a mental picture that you can revisit whenever you want.

You could also try making belly dance, salsa, or hula-hoop-like movements with your body while standing upright, where the focus should be on moving your abdomen in a circular or side-to-side motion. This may feel as though you are stirring yourself up, but this is how you will be unblocking any trapped energy. By placing two fingers just below your navel, begin to move them slowly in a clockwise (female) or counterclockwise (male) motion. This will raise sensations in your sacral chakra and activate your sensual feelings. You may notice a gentle pulsing, but if you don't notice this immediately, you may want to try this a few more times when your energy is centered on the feeling within rather than the movement of the fingers.

An important tip to note is to try not to overdo this practice at one go. You certainly wouldn't want to start feeling discomfort or an ache in your belly since this will be the complete opposite of what you are meant to achieve. This may also leave your sacral chakra unbalanced. When the energy you feel has passed through the other chakras, you may calm yourself by taking gentle breaths to relieve or release any tightness and residual energy that might have built up from this practice. You should caution against rushing the progress of any of your chakra balancing practices since this could result in causing strain to your life force energy.

A few ideas that you could consider are painting, drawing, or craftwork. Painting and drawing are mental workouts of having fun while doing something that helps you liberate a picture that might only be trapped in your mind. When you express yourself this way, you may also note the choice of colors you use, any patterns or inconsistencies in whatever is being drawn or painted, or any feelings and sensations you experience while doing this. If you are considering craftwork, you could look at options such as pottery or beadwork since these are also good techniques for balancing and unblocking the sacral chakra.

I have found that walking through the park with my headphones on while listening to shamanic drumming music is very helpful for placing my awareness into my sacral chakra. In one instance, I realized that the drumming is rhythmic, pounding, and has deep tones that make my feet want to thump freely on the ground as I walk. Sometimes, I simply let them. My intention is to shift some unknown stagnate energy from my creative center.

While walking, thoughts of how I have had a nagging feeling to create but haven't found the motivation to do so during the last few days were rushing at me. I knew this was a blockage because creativity flows naturally when the energy is freely moving through the sacral chakra. When the desire to create flows naturally, it's fun and seemingly spontaneous—just the way I like it. As I kept walking, I would take in some new energy through breathing into my sacral chakra. I would imagine an orange light coming into my mouth and entering my being to settle in between my hips. I would relax this area and allow it the freedom to sway and move as I walk.

It would almost resemble belly dancing since I could feel the rise and fall of my hips going up and down to the drums. I would feel the swirls of my belly with each thump. The music grew intoxicating. I could feel the sensuality of the music and my body, and I openly allowed this feeling to fill my awareness. As I continued to walk, flashes of new inspiration came to my awareness. This was how I knew that my chakra energies were reawakening. After a few magical, sensual laps of the drumming rhythms and walking around my circuit, I sat down on a park bench and allowed my awareness to go to my sacral chakra.

While seated, I closed my eyes and began to feel into this space, and I could see orange. It was quite vibrant and seemed to have its own identity. Once I opened my eyes, I could see a multitude of birds pecking in the grass in front of me. For a moment, I would glimpse at their sacral chakras and smile to myself. I was pondering on the thought that they, too, are energy and that we are ultimately connected. In my mind's eye, I could see an orange cord connecting all their sacral chakras, including my own. This orange cord was like a glowing orange network of light connecting us all. On my way back home, I unplugged and allowed myself space to be. All sorts of ideas and inspirations flowed easily to my mind's eye. I could see that working my sacral energies this way clears the canvas for new inspirations to flow.

So, you might want to start making a habit of clearing your mind as often as possible to ensure that you aren't hindering the flow of creativity and sensuality. After all, you are the only person responsible for this mental clearance. Imagine if someone else bore the responsibility to get you geared into mental focus every time it drifted away. Do you think that person would contribute positively to your mental development while also tending to their mental needs? I strongly doubt that. So, realize the importance of taking charge of your mind space to enhance your power, and you will start to see the benefits pour into how you easily clear up any clutter from your life. The importance of being responsible for your well-being through your chakra balancing will be discussed a little more in the next chapter, with a focus on the solar plexus chakra.

Chapter 5

THE CROWN CHAKRA: YOUR COSMIC PORTAL

Location and Physical Association
Let's venture to the very top of your head, where babies have a soft spot. This is the location of your seventh chakra, the Crown Chakra, known as *Sahasrara* in Sanskrit. This chakra is associated with the top of the head, the brain, and the entire nervous system. It also governs the pineal gland, which is known to secrete the hormone melatonin, regulating sleep and wakefulness.

Emotional and Spiritual Significance
The Crown Chakra is your spiritual antenna, your cosmic portal to the divine. It's your spiritual Wi-Fi, connecting you with the universe and the divine energy that flows through it. When your Crown Chakra is balanced, you feel a deep sense of peace and a connection with the universe. It's

like being tuned into a cosmic radio station, receiving divine wisdom and understanding.
This chakra is also associated with enlightenment and self-realization. It's about transcending the physical and the individual to connect with the collective consciousness. With a balanced Crown Chakra, you experience a sense of wonder and awe for the interconnectedness of all life and the mystery of existence.

Common Imbalances
When the Crown Chakra is out of balance, it's like losing the Wi-Fi signal and being disconnected from the cosmic web. Physically, you might experience headaches, light sensitivity, or neurological disorders.
Emotionally, you might feel disconnected or isolated, like you've lost your sense of belonging in the universe. You might also experience a

spiritual crisis, question the meaning and purpose of life, or experience a loss of faith.

On the other hand, an overactive Crown Chakra might manifest as an obsession with spirituality to the detriment of your physical needs. You might neglect your bodily needs, become ungrounded, or have difficulty living in the real world.

Healing Techniques

So, how do you realign your Crown Chakra and restore your cosmic connection? Here are some techniques:

Meditation: Since the Crown Chakra is all about spiritual connection, meditation is one of the most effective practices to balance this chakra. You can focus on your breath or use a mantra, like I am connected with the divine.

Silence: Spending time in silence can help open up your Crown Chakra. It's like turning down the world's noise to hear the universe's whispers.

Fasting or detox: Periodically giving your body a break from digesting food can help stimulate the Crown Chakra. Always consult with a healthcare provider before starting a fast or detox.

Crystals: Clear or violet crystals like selenite or amethyst can help balance the Crown Chakra.

Aromatherapy: Essential oils like frankincense or myrrh can help stimulate the Crown Chakra and enhance your spiritual connection.

So there we have it, the Crown Chakra, your cosmic portal, linking you with the universe and the divine energy that flows through it. By nurturing this chakra, you can cultivate a deep sense of awe, wonder, and connection with all that is. You become a part of the cosmic dance, moving with the universe's rhythm, guided by the melody of divine wisdom. So, tune into your Crown Chakra and dance away, my friend! The cosmic dance floor awaits.

SCIENTIFIC DEMONSTRATION OF THE ENERGY FIELD

For a more detailed reading, I recommend the texts written directly by Prof. Vinardi; you will find a complete list at the end of this book. My aim is merely to present an introductory summary of his unique research on the human aura, so as to lead the reader to a deeper understanding of the extraordinary knowledge transmitted by the Professor. To mention just one, the BPE, the discipline he founded, consists of four volumes, the last of which concerning Biorhythmology, is a true didactic, critical, comparative treatise on vital rhythms: more than 500 pages of pure science. A work of extraordinary value. It is therefore understandable that this text will only serve for the dissemination of elementary concepts and as an introduction to a subject that, ultimately, has to do with self-knowledge.

To scientifically demonstrate the existence of the human aura, Vinardi worked with a coil made up of different elements such as copper-bronze-aluminum, capable of containing a lying person within it. In his books, you can see photos of these electromagnetic coils in action, i.e., with a patient inside, about 2 meters long with a diameter between 60 and 80 centimeters.

The coil was part of a circuit that was integrated with various laboratory instruments such as: polygraph, oscilloscope, assymeter, phase meter, tester, wave modulators and generators, and the Q-meter. The latter in electrical engineering and electronics is called quality factor and is used to measure the resonance coefficient of a circuit. It is used to evaluate this factor in coils, radio resonant circuits, and more. Prof. Vinardi measured the Q factor of the person housed in the coil, which was subject to a variety of different stimuli, such as biomagnets, chromoenergetics, infra and ultrasounds, low and high-frequency radio wave generators, homeopathy, acupuncture, etc.

The bioplasmic field weighting project included a total of 38 programs and 10,459 measurements, over a span of ten years.

Even though a photographic objectification of the human aura, albeit limited, was obtained with Kirlian photography, Vinardi chose the coil to carry out his research, starting from the base of a General Theory of Living Systems, according to the BPE he founded: the evident movement and development in a vortex form of everything that appears in the physical universe observed, from DNA to the galaxy to which our sun belongs, from the movement of subatomic particles to swirls, tides, tsunamis, and tornadoes. A common thread that allowed to observe the same configuration in the human energy field and thus offer the appropriate tools to reach certain measurements.

Going into more detail: if I take a coil, an element found in many household objects, and measure its values, it will give me a result corresponding to the unit that corresponds to it. If it contains nothing, therefore with an empty core, or if I put materials such as a piece of cloth, paper, or wood inside it, by measuring it I will notice that its value does not change, and this by virtue of the fact that they are not conductive materials, but insulating ones. If, on the other hand, I put a piece of iron inside, I will notice that there is a reaction and therefore a difference between a measurement made with an empty core and one with iron. I could even observe a difference depending on whether the iron is powdered or laminated. Vinardi used a human being as the core of the coil to verify whether certain discharges were actually produced, like a current generator; very subtle discharges, which the coil receives in the form of influences that translate into different values and that are reported by the Q factor meter.

Since the coil and the core are a single complex, it was possible to modify the behavior of the core, through the use of biomagnets, or even through deep breaths, or certain types of concentration of the core itself, and by using mathematical models, some interpretations of the data obtained were reached. What Vinardi wanted to measure was in fact the space between the person lying inside the coil and the coil itself. A space that, without any extrasensory perception, might seem empty, but is not. That space is full and has been the subject of measurements with the stimuli already mentioned. Vinardi, to give other examples, also used colored light sources, i.e., bulbs from the simplest to the most sophisticated (ultraviolet and also infrared lamps) to study the influences of wavelengths on the space between the person and the coil. As I already said, 38 programs were developed. It was thus seen that these external stimuli act in some way, as mechanical or electromagnetic waves, producing just those changes that were of interest.

The conclusion of the studies carried out at San Francisco State University was to confirm the existence of a measurable field that is not only found outside the skin but also inside. This is because the living nervous system, inside a living body with its trillions of cells, creates bioelectricity and therefore a discreet energy field.

Biology and medicine study the human being organically from the skin inward, but the personal continent is much larger than that described by these important sciences.

To date (year 2021), as far as I know, no one has ever produced such extensive documentation of scientific evidence and such a complete exposition on the existence of the Human Energy Field or as it is called by the Russian and American schools, respectively Biological Organizer Model – MOB – or Bioplasmic Field. Names that are added to others that have followed over the course of history, such as:

etheric double, according to Theosophy;

N-ray, or odic force, according to Reichenbach;

perispirit, according to spiritualists;

psychotronic field, according to the Russians during the period of the Soviet Union and finally Human Aura.

Below are the material and scientific foundations of physical order that will facilitate the links and define the conclusions on the next topics.

Chapter 6

Muladhara

The term Muladhara finds its roots in Mool and Aadhar, signifying Prime and Foundation respectively. True to its name, Muladhara represents the bedrock of the human body's existence. This chakra, painted in vibrant hues of red, serves as the cornerstone for various physical activities. Aligned with the trilogy of the lower chakras, Muladhara intertwines with the essential aspects of the physical self. It is the epicenter of the body's foundational energy, symbolizing the vitality and force that propels all manners of physical endeavors. Muladhara's significance lies in its role as the grounding force, anchoring the human experience in the realm of the physical. If Muladhara is strengthened any kind of fear leaves the body and nothing supernatural affects the body at all. If one's energy is rooted properly in Muladhara the person will find himself constantly hungry. The metabolism of such a person is very high and they do not have any stomach-related issues. It might be considered a coincidence, however, it is not, as the human body grows old, more stomach-related issues arise, that is because the body's expiry date is nearing and Muladhara is weakening. But if your age is young and you still have stomach-related issues, and a week Muladhara, it indicates the past-lives karma or heavy karmic debt, which is yet to be unfolded or solved and it is advised for you to start now.

If the Muladhara is affected to the very core of the destruction of one's physical form (which essentially means if you have been in any kind of physical traumatic situation or accident) then it is advised never to sleep in the pure dark. You should have at least a lamp lighting in your room, any kind of vegetable oil can be used. If a lamp is taking too much effort or it is not possible, then light a small bulb, but a pure dark situation will not let your Muladhara rest while you think you are asleep.

Muladhara is the basic foundation which also indicates its links with earth elements. A distressed Muladhara can easily be fixed with 21 minutes of chanting of LUM mantra or by 30 minutes of grounding with bare feet walking at the earth's surface. One can also try gardening or if nothing of this is possible, please take some soil from your garden or from anywhere (some temple soil is recommended) and just apply it on the arc of your feet. (If possible you can add the other auspicious material as well like Gaumutra or drops of Gangajal.) Also the chanting of Aum is recommended for such an individual.

Now this may seem superficial but wearing undergarments either washed totally in soil or of colour red is recommended for strengthening a very ditoriating Muladhara. The goddess Kamalatmika is believed to reside in Muladhara and she is also considered as Maha-Lakshami, so worshipping her will fairly help you recover from distorted Muladhara.

Chapter 7

Open Your Root Chakra with Yoga

The chakra responsible for those physical energies that provide us the sense of security and satisfaction is the root chakra or muladhara. Out of the seven chakras, this one is located at the base of an individual's spine. Muladhara, as per Hindu tantrism, is a combination of two Sanskrit words i.e. Mula- root and Adhara-base.

By balancing the root chakra, a strong base is created for opening the other chakras. Strengthening of this chakra is similar to the establishment of the framework for a house in which you're going to live for an extensive period of time. A strong foundation in a firm soil will provide the strength and ability to create a home loaded with joy and satisfaction for future.

The root chakra is composed of all those things which keep you intact with stability in your life. These things include your lower order needs such as food, shelter, water, and security. Moreover, those emotional needs that control your behavior are also part of this chakra. Interestingly, when these needs are fulfilled, you feel secure and your fear starts diminishing.

Kundalini power is put away here, change can happen when these energies are excited and permitted to ascend inside you and enter each Chakra above. The vitality joins the Shakti vitality at the Heart Center, proceeds on and leaves the body through the highest point of the head - or Crown Chakra. As this happens, profound development and familiarity with different levels of vitality and observations happen.

However, these feelings of safety and security are clearly more dependent on how you felt in your childhood rather than what you feel or possess today. A psychological insight can be used to expound upon the root chakra. As per Erik Ericson's stages of development, first stage i.e. trust versus mistrust, has a close proximity with this base chakra. If an infant is provided with care and love, he develops the feeling that this world and the people here can be trusted. However, if he is not provided with enough care then adverse feelings are imprinted on the infant's mind for the rest of his life. You might feel blockages in the first chakra if you had experienced the latter case.

Disparity in Root Chakra:

Disparity in this chakra might result in multiple psychological disorders. A few of these psychological problems are listed as follows:

- Nightmares
- Anxiety
- Phobias

Other physical imbalances that might result include eating disorders, lower back, leg, and feet issues.

Healing the Disparities of Root Chakra:

To begin with, disparities in this chakra can cause several problems both on psychological and physical level. Therefore, one must adopt those activities that will heal these problems. Multiple approaches that are used for healing purposes are as follow

Assertion of the Root Chakra:

This technique is a sound therapy in which settles with his/her presence in this world. It usually comprises an assertion by an individual that this place is safe for me. I belong here. Moreover, the person further states that I am in peace with the people and events around me.

- Color Therapy:

The color therapy has an association with red color. An individual has to imagine a red lotus right at the base of spine where the root chakra is located. This process of picturing the flower can help in balancing the chakra. Light a few candles to have better consequences.

Other activities that are adopted by people to balance this chakra include the use of crystals, oil and sound. However, one of the most eminent techniques to eliminate the disparity of root chakra is yoga.

Yoga as an Opening Tool for Root Chakra:

Yoga is a physical as well as a spiritual practice which is not only an exercise for your body but also it is an efficacious tool to refresh your mind, emotions and spirit. Hence, it is one of the perfect practices in order to balance the imbalanced chakra. Of all the postures those poses are most efficient which create connection with the motherly plant-Earth.

Following are some yoga poses to open your root chakra:

Mountain pose-Tadasana:

Tadasana also known as mountain pose is one of the most simple and common poses of yoga. All yoga practitioners began their journey with this easy pose. The advantage of this pose is its ability to connect the practitioner with earth. Moreover, this connection helps you in grounding yourself. This pose is loved by everyone because it makes an individual calmer and relaxed.

Procedure:

Firstly, stand on your yoga mat. Keep your shoulders tight and straight. Your chin must be parallel with the surface. Keep your arms at side. Focus on your breath. Now start breathing slowly. Inhale the air into your belly through your head and let the lungs contract. Now relax, and exhale. Keep doing this again and again.

Now start feeling the ground under your feet. Lift your toes up, inhale and then exhale by putting your feet back on the mat

You will start feeling grounded by imagining the connection between you and the ground. This will bring stability and strength

Keep on doing the practice till you feel like standing strong as a mountain. This technique surely balances your chakra.

Warrior One Pose-Virabhadrasana 1:

This posture is an amazing asana since it creates a firm association between you and the earth. This root chakra yoga posture permits your prana to travel through your body. Consequently, your root chakra will be balanced. This pose also strengthens a person physically.

Procedure:

Stand straight in mountain pose. Take a full breath and, while exhaling, stride your left foot back around 3.5 feet.

Turn your left foot to around a 45-degree edge. Make sure your left foot is immovably planted and touching the ground.

While you exhale, twist your right knee over the right lower leg, so that your shin is opposite to the floor. In the event that you can, carry your right thigh parallel with the floor.

- Raise your arms over your head and touch the palms together

Inhale profoundly and hold the position for one moment.

- Twist your knees and step your feet back together. Now repeat this posture on the other side

Bridge Pose-Setu Bhandasana

This posture is dynamic root chakra yoga pose. This posture permits your feet to be immovably established into the Earth and your spine occupied with the arrival of overabundance root chakra vitality.

Procedure:

To begin with, lay on your back with your arms straight close by, palms confronting down.

Twist your knees and keep your feet parallel to each other, about hip-width separated.

Convey your heels near your body with the goal that you can feel the tips of your fingers.

While keeping up full contact with the ground, press your feet into the mat. Connect with your leg muscles, yet don't lift yourself up. Feel the vitality coursing through your legs. Inhale profoundly.

Press your feet significantly more and lift your bum and your lower back off the ground. Press the mid-section upward.

You can bolster yourself in this position with your hands by setting them on your lower back. Inhale gradually and equally and hold the posture for one moment.

Chapter 8

Chakras' Teachings:

A Path to Life Transformation.

Chakras' Wisdom: Attracting Abundance weaves life's invaluable lessons into the energy centers of transformation, where holistic well-being, prosperity, and abundance await the awakened soul.

The concept of energy fields has a long history in Eastern cultures, where health, medicine and life are defined in relation to the flow of energy. More recently, such concepts have begun to be incorporated in Western cultures into theories of health and healing within medicine. Human energy fields exist within the body and around the body, with specific energy centers called chakras.

The knowledge of chakras is very ancient and was mentioned by the Vedas more than 5,000 years ago. The knowledge of everything in life is included in each of the chakras of the human body, where the seven of them are the gauges of human life. Each of the seven major chakras in our body represents different dimensions of our life.

They take positive energy from the environment to keep us physically, mentally and emotionally healthy. And if these chakras are closed for some reason, they stop receiving positive energy from the environment and begin to bring physical illnesses, emotional conflicts and problems in life in general.

Here's a simplified explanation of how the chakras are often thought to interact with energy for overall well-being:

Receiving energy: The chakras are considered to be receivers of energy, both from the external environment and from within our own being. These energy centers act like vortexes, drawing in vital energy.

Processing energy: Once the chakras receive energy, they are thought to process it. Different chakras are associated with specific qualities and attributes. Each chakra processes energy related to its associated qualities.

Balancing and distributing Energy: The chakras balance and distribute energy throughout the body. This balance is thought to contribute to overall physical, mental, and emotional well-being.

Imbalances and health issues: Imbalances or blockages in the chakras disrupt the flow of energy, potentially leading to physical or emotional health issues.

The chakras described in this book are seven subtle energy centers within the human body, which emit cosmic frequencies to create perfect harmony between mind, body and soul. Located along the spine, at the points where nerve plexuses converge and endocrine glands are located, these invisible centers are valves that regulate the flow of universal energy through our energy system. The chakras govern every aspect of our lives: expressions, feelings and senses – even the sixth sense.

The chakras create balanced physical, mental and emotional health when they are functioning at their best. However, as you go through experiences and challenges in life, whenever your thoughts, attitudes and reactions tend towards fear or negativity, your chakras get blocked. With a blockage in the chakras, the free flow of cosmic energy in the body is inhibited. At this point, you begin to develop emotional disorders and physical ailments related to the chakras.

For the chakras to open again, you must release these blocked emotions and let go of your limiting beliefs and rigid, dogmatic perceptions. By working with your chakras, you eliminate stagnant negative energy that does not serve your highest purpose. Doing this will broaden your perspective, aid in your evolution as a human being, and help you make the changes necessary to improve your health, harmonious relationships, and personal and financial well-being.

Ancient yogic wisdom emphasized the connection between physical, mental and spiritual health in human beings. This connection between body, mind and spirit is enabled by the cosmic energy centers in our body. These energy centers are called chakras. The Sanskrit word chakra means wheel or disc. One can visualize the chakras as rotating vortices or wheels of cosmic energy, where matter meets life force, chi, ki or prana. Our body contains seven major chakras, whose specific positions throughout our body correspond with extensive nerve centers and major endocrine glands. The seven chakras are located along the spine, from the tailbone to the crown of the head. These subtle energy centers absorb and distribute vital energy throughout the body so that there is proper flow of energy to and from all body parts and vital organs. The seven main chakras take care of specific parts and organs of the body.

All of our body's chakras must be open, in alignment, and in motion for our general well-being. Every disruption or obstruction prevents the free life force energy from flowing, which is essential for the evolution of every cell in the body. The way our mind, thoughts, emotions, perceptions, and even our sixth sense work are all directly related to how the chakras function. The chakras are seen as a vital part of the mind-body-spirit connection and play a significant role in shaping our consciousness and experiences.

Here's a closer look at how chakras are thought to relate to various aspects of our mental and emotional well-being:

Mind and Thoughts: Each chakra is associated with specific psychological and cognitive qualities. For example, the crown chakra is connected to higher consciousness and understanding, while the third eye chakra is linked to intuition and insight. When the chakras are balanced and open, it is believed that mental clarity and thought processes can function optimally. Imbalances in the chakras might result in mental fogginess, negative thought patterns, or difficulty in decision-making.

Emotions: The chakras also have emotional attributes. For instance, the heart chakra is associated with love, compassion, and forgiveness, while the sacral chakra relates to emotions, sensuality, and creativity. Balancing and harmonizing the chakras is thought to help regulate and promote emotional wellbeing.

Perceptions: The chakras influence our perceptions of the world and how we interpret experiences. For example, the throat chakra is connected to honest and clear communication, which can shape how we perceive and interpret information. A balanced throat chakra is thought to enhance our ability to express our thoughts and to perceive things with clarity.

Intuition (Sixth Sense): The concept of a sixth sense or intuition is associated with the third eye chakra, which is the seat of inner knowing and psychic abilities. A balanced and open third eye chakra is said to sharpen intuition and insight. The energy of the chakras change whenever our thoughts, attitudes, and behaviors lean toward fear or negativity. Depending on the thought pattern and type of rigidly held limiting beliefs, the chakras can become overactive, underactive, or completely blocked. With a blockage in the chakras, the free flow of cosmic energy in the body is inhibited. This is how the chakras establish the mind-body connection. Healthy and balanced chakras are the key to holistic health and well-being on a physical, emotional and spiritual level.

We must realize that life provides for us in a variety of ways and that it continually creates new things such as plants, knowledge, technology, etc. And what we have to do is tune in and align ourselves with life. And thus understand the laws and life lessons through the chakras. If we abide by these laws and lessons, which are completely under our control, we will have all the benefits that life has to offer us. Human beings don't like to be constrained or limited in any manner. And we exert every effort to achieve limitlessness. However, what blocks us from being limitless is in the seven major chakras.

First, in order to self-realize, self-recognize, or be aware of our limitless potential, we must walk through the laws and lessons of the seven chakras. And in order to do this, we must become one with life. This is known as enlightenment.

The seven primary chakras, or subtle energy centers, are present in every living thing. These centers represent the seven aspects of awareness or the seven dimensions of human life. These chakras are situated along the spinal column's network of veins, arteries, and nerves.

Chakras function as receivers and transformers of various types of energy that flow in a spiral pattern as long as they are open. Five of these chakras are on both sides of the body; front and backside. What we receive from the world is on the backside of our body while what we give to the world is on the front side. Therefore, we cannot limit our desires to receiving since in order to receive, one must first give. You must show love if you expect to receive it. You must support others if you expect them to do the same for you. You must accept yourself if you want other people to accept you. If you want people to trust you, you have to trust both people and life.

All these chakras have distinctive colors and stand for various energies. And the ancient sages taught us that each chakra has certain laws and lessons to impart.

Therefore, the Root Chakra (Muladhara) is located in the position of the adrenal glands, whose function is to fight or flight. This chakra is guiding you to realize what causes instabilities, emotional loss, financial loss and other related issues. You will also learn about the fears that have unbalanced this chakra. Learn the lessons to attract Support and Stability in life. You will learn the Root Chakra's Law: You have the right to be and have support and stability, because you were born and you are life itself.

The Sacral chakra (Swadhisthana) is located two inches below the navel and is in the position of the gonad glands: the ovaries and testicles, the organs of reproduction. We also name it the sexuality chakra. It is guiding you to realize what causes emotional immaturity, inability to adapt to changes, depression, mood swings, sexual dysfunctions and other related problems. You will also learn about the fears that have unbalanced this chakra. Learn the lessons so you can realize your unique identity. You will learn the Sacral Chakra's Law: You are unique and special. You build your self-esteem by honoring your identity. The Solar Plexus Chakra (Manipura) is located in the pit of the stomach and is related to the pancreas, which governs digestion and gastric juices. This is guiding you towards understanding the type of expectations, incorrect definitions, dependency issues and other related issues that unbalance this chakra. You will also learn about the fears that have unbalanced this chakra. Learn the lessons so that you realize how you can be Powerful and Independent. You will learn the Solar Plexus Chakra's Law: You are powerful and independent. You can do all tasks with grace and ease.

The Heart Chakra (Anahata) is related to the thymus gland. And regulate the rhythms. This is guiding you towards understanding past negative references and self-destructive tendencies that have unbalanced this chakra. You will also learn about the fears that have further unbalanced this chakra. Learn the lessons so you realize how you can begin to love and manifest everything you truly desire. You will learn the Heart Chakra's Law: You are a creator. You are a divine being who can manifest your desires.

The Throat Chakra (Vishuddha) is located at the level of the pit of the throat and is related to the thyroid glands: thyroid and parathyroid. This chakra is guiding you toward understanding the knowledge gaps you have created in your life and the related comparison tendencies that have unbalanced this chakra. You will also learn about the fears that have most unbalanced this chakra. Learn the lessons so that you realize and establish your Knowledge and Wisdom to express yourself perfectly. You will learn the Throat Chakra's Law: You are an effective communicator. You are full of knowledge and wisdom.

The Third Eye Chakra (Ajna) is located between the eyebrows and is related to the pituitary gland. This chakra is guiding you to see the falsehood, the illusions, the acceptance problems and the fears that have caused the imbalance of this chakra. Learn the lessons so that you can realize your Higher Intelligence that helps you make right decisions. You will learn the Third Eye Chakra's Law: You are intuitive and wise. You make healthy decisions with your higher intelligence.

And the Crown Chakra (Sahasrara) is located in the crown of the head and is related to the pineal gland. This chakra guides you to realize how discontent and related problems, how certain types of fears and isolation can block your connection with the Universe, thus blocking your power to access abundance and unbalancing this chakra. Learn the lessons so you can create Abundance in every aspect of your life. You will learn the Crown Chakra's Law: You are fortunate and abundant. You align with your true nature through gratitude and satisfaction.

Scientists and neurochemists have shown that disorders in the body can result from problems with any of these endocrine glands, which are closely related to the chakras. Problems with your root chakra will affect your entire skeletal system. You will experience problems with your entire muscle system if your sacral chakra is not functioning properly. Your digestive system will function improperly if the Solar Plexus chakra is out of balance.

You will have issues with your circulatory system, heart, lungs, and skin if your heart chakra is out of balance. You will have thyroid problems, sleep issues, and hair loss if your throat chakra is out of balance. You will have sinus issues and headaches if your brow third-eye chakra is out of balance. Additionally, if your Crown chakra is not functioning properly, you will experience nerve problems, paralysis, and migraines.

Each chakra's laws and lessons about everything affecting your life may be learned and recognized as part of the process of healing the chakras. Nowadays doctors tell you that if you want to cure a disease, you must eliminate stress. And stress is eliminated when you heal your thoughts and the way you perceive life situations. Stress is not solely caused by external events or circumstances but is closely tied to the way we think and perceive life situations.

Managing stress often involves addressing and reshaping our thought patterns, perspectives, and reactions to various stressors. If you are stressed because your career is not going well, you will only be permanently healed when you learn to handle that situation, when you realize that you have the knowledge and the power to handle that situation. This is how you remove and release stress with wisdom.

Your chakras will teach you how to handle situations spiritually. The secret to overcoming obstacles is to study and know the natural laws and life teachings inherent in each of the seven main chakras. You are now living in fear and misery as a result of your ignorance of the laws and teachings that govern your existence. The instant you realize them, you are prepared for what will occur and are aware of how to handle it.

Being conscious of oneself eliminates the need for fear of potential outcomes. But why do individuals have so many fears? What if my health worsens, What if I lose the money, What if my family suffers, What if I lose my job or my business, etc. Because you are unaware of the laws and lessons governing your life through the chakras.

You will become peaceful, kind, and friendly if you are aware of the laws, lights, and lessons governing daily life. According to Proverbs 16:15 in the Bible, When a king's face brightens, it means life; his favor is like a rain cloud in spring, you will be peaceful. That is to say, you will not be present and you will not be able to remain calm and unshakable as long as you have many thoughts fluttering in your mind, flying around like birds without a nest. Enlightenment arrives when you are present, calm, and unshakable.

It is useful to learn these guidelines or teachings from the chakras in order to heal them. According to this approach, healing entails understanding the teachings of each chakra and being prepared to handle challenging circumstances to avoid suffering. Learning from the teachings of the chakras can indeed be a valuable path to healing and personal growth. Here's how this approach works:

Chakra teachings: Each chakra is believed to impart specific life lessons, attributes, and qualities.

Self-Reflection: To heal and balance the chakras, individuals engage in self-reflection and self-awareness. They explore their beliefs, emotions, and thought patterns in the context of the teachings associated with each chakra.

Identifying challenges: By understanding the teachings of the chakras, individuals can identify areas of their lives where they may be facing challenges or experiencing imbalances. These challenges may be related to the qualities associated with specific chakras.

Resolving challenges: The teachings of the chakras provide guidance on how to resolve these challenges. For example, if one is facing difficulties related to self-esteem and personal power (solar plexus chakra), the chakra's teachings can guide them toward building self-confidence and assertiveness.

Preventing suffering: The ultimate goal is to use this knowledge to avoid unnecessary suffering. By aligning one's life with the teachings of the chakras, individuals aim to live in harmony, make more conscious choices, and respond to life's challenges with resilience and wisdom.

Holistic healing: The approach recognizes that healing is a holistic process, addressing not only physical symptoms but also emotional, mental, and spiritual well-being.

Chapter 9

Some of the life lessons of the Seven Major Chakras:

Our entire relationship with life is about bringing light to our darkness.
You are tuned into the nature of life by each chakra. Nothing should limit you. You have to go from darkness into light. And in order to do it you must abide by your divine law, your light:
In your darkness you feel unsupported and insecure. However, you have to go towards your light, which tells you that you are divinely supported and stable because it is your nature to have stability. The Root Chakra (Muladhara) teaches you to honor your parents, work and your body, and synchronizes you with hard work, honoring unity and dealing with life's challenges. This basically evokes the warrior in you and tells

you that you are here to stay, that you have the right to exist because you exist, you were born. And to synchronize yourself with this chakra, it tells you to release the fear of survival.

In your darkness you are feeling an identity crisis and have personal doubts. However, when you decide to move into your light, your divine nature, tells you that you are special, creative and unique. The Sacral Chakra (Swadhisthana) teaches you how to honor yourself and others. It says that you are here because life is realizing, updating or recognizing you through one of its forms. You can say that you are the Supreme Being incarnate, who is here to give you that challenge, which is also a way of life. Therefore, it tells you to release the fear that people might take advantage of you. In your darkness you feel powerless and victimized, but once you discover your light, you realize that you are powerful and independent because your nature is to be powerful. The Solar

Plexus Chakra (Manipura) teaches you to honor your opinions and internalize or go inward. Likewise to honor the opinions of others and direct them. Since only then will you have the power of action to transform your environment. To do this, it tells you to release the fear of dependency and the feelings of victimization associated with dependency.

In your darkness you feel distrustful of your dreams and desires, without realizing such light within you that tells you that you are a creator, since that is your nature, creation. The Heart Chakra (Anahata) teaches you to synchronize with unconditional love and trust, as well as selfless giving. And for that, it tells you to release the fears of mistrust and the expectations of others. In your darkness you have difficulties with understanding and being understood. However, your true nature, your divine light is that you are an effective communicator. The Throat Chakra

(Vishuddha) teaches you to synchronize with your nature of expression and understanding. And for that, it tells you to release fears of comparison with others.

In your darkness you feel indecisive and have difficulty accepting what IS. However, when you realize that your divine nature is to be wise and intelligent, you turn to the light within you that tells you that you are intuitive and wise. The Third Eye Chakra (Ajna) teaches you to accept what IS, the Truth, the Reality. And for that, it tells you to release the definitions and false perceptions or beliefs through which you identify with the world from the lens of your egoic Self.

In your darkness you feel hopeless, dissatisfied and disconnected. However, when you recognize the divine light that is in you, which tells you that you are fortunate and abundant, you realize that you no longer want to live in dissatisfaction and scarcity because your nature is to be abundant.

The Crown Chakra (Sahasrara) teaches you to synchronize with contentment and gratitude. And for that, it says to free yourself from hopelessness, dissatisfaction and limiting beliefs. When the nature of life is survival in the Root Chakra, creativity in the Sacral Chakra, power in the Solar Plexus Chakra, love in the Heart Chakra, expression in the Throat Chakra, truth in the Third Eye Chakra, and abundance in the Chakra Corona, do you think life could destroy you? No, because life is Mother, who nourishes and cares. Have faith and trust. Life created you and will take care of you at every moment. It gives you power to resolve anything that comes to you. It gives you all the experiences that make you develop your Higher Self. It has given you wisdom and intelligence. All you need to do is let yourself be guided by the teachings or lessons that life gives you through the chakras.

Let's look in depth at what those life lessons contained in each of the seven major chakras teach us.

Chakras' wisdom and life lessons intertwine at the crossroads of energy centers, forging a path towards the harmonious unity of mind, body, and spirit, and along this journey unfolds the gateway to holistic well-being, prosperity, and limitless abundance.

Embracing the profound chakras' life lessons is the path to self-realization, unlocking your true nature and inviting boundless abundance into every facet of your existence. From the foundational right to support and stability in the first chakra, to the nurturing of self-esteem in the second, the empowerment and grace in the third, the creative manifestation of desires in the fourth, the wisdom and knowledge in the fifth, the intuitive and healthy decisions in the sixth, to finally aligning with your true nature and experiencing gratitude and satisfaction in the seventh – these chakras' teachings are the keys to a life enriched by abundance, harmony, and self-discovery.

CHAPTER 10

THE PRIMARY SEVEN CHAKRAS

Muladhara, The Root Chakra:

At the base of the spine is the basic energy point known as the Root Chakra, or Muladhara. It stands for our rootedness in the material world, which provides us with stability and security. This chakra, represented by the color red, is linked to survival instincts, fundamental necessities, and a sense of community.

People who have a balanced Root Chakra experience a great sense of security and stability. Exercises that balance and stimulate the Root Chakra, such as yoga positions, meditation, and grounding techniques, can help build a strong foundation for personal development.

Svadhisthana, the sacral chakra:

As we ascend the spine, the Sacral Chakra, also known as the Svadhisthana, is located directly below the navel. The creative process, sensuality, and emotional stability are associated with this chakra. It is symbolized by the color orange and is in charge of our capacity for enjoyment and close relationships. One experiences an abundance of creativity and a healthy outlet for their emotions when the Sacral Chakra is in balance. This chakra can be regulated by being creative, expressing emotions, and engaging in mindfulness exercises.

Manipura's solar plexus chakra:
 The Solar Plexus Chakra, also known as Manipura, is situated in the upper belly and is linked to self-worth, confidence, and personal strength. This yellow chakra affects our sense of self and independence.

An ability to pursue goals with determination and a strong sense of self-worth are the results of a balanced Solar Plexus Chakra. The Solar Plexus Chakra can be balanced and activated with the use of techniques like mindful breathing, core-strengthening exercises, and positive affirmations.

Anahata, The Heart Chakra:

The Heart Chakra, also known as Anahata, is located in the middle of the chest and serves as the center for emotional equilibrium, love, and compassion. It is represented by the color green and controls our ability to love ourselves and others. People who have a balanced Heart Chakra report having harmonious relationships and a strong bond with all living things.

The Heart Chakra is balanced by engaging in activities like loving-kindness meditation, heart-opening yoga poses, and deeds of compassion.

The Vishuddha Chakra (throat):

Moving on to the throat area, the Throat Chakra, also known as Vishuddha, is connected to self-expression, communication, and genuineness. This chakra, symbolized by the color blue, affects one's capacity for honest and clear thought and emotional expression. A healthy throat chakra encourages clear communication and the guts to tell it like it is. Throat Chakra can be balanced and activated by singing, saying affirmations, and doing throat-opening yoga positions.

Ajna, the Third Eye Chakra:

The Third Eye Chakra, also known as Ajna, is located in the forehead between the eyebrows and is associated with spiritual insight, awareness, and intuition. It is indigo in color and represents the core of higher consciousness and inner wisdom. People who have a balanced Third Eye Chakra report having better intuition and a stronger sense of inner connection. This chakra is aligned in part by third eye stimulation, meditation, and visualization techniques.

Sahasrara, The Crown Chakra

The doorway to higher stages of awareness and spiritual consciousness is the Crown Chakra, also known as Sahasrara, located at the crown of the head. This chakra, which is symbolized by the colors violet or white, ties us to the energy of the universe and the divine. One experiences transcendence, bliss, and unity when their Crown Chakra is balanced. Praying, meditation, and mindfulness exercises all help to align and activate the Crown Chakra.

Chakra Alignment And Balancing:

Chakra alignment and balance are essential for general health and optimal energy flow. This balance can be attained through a variety of activities, such as energy healing methods, yoga, meditation, and breathwork. Through meditation, people can concentrate on each chakra, releasing obstructions and reestablishing equilibrium. Chakra-specific yoga poses facilitate the release of tension and encourage the flow of energy. In addition, energy healing techniques like Reiki and mindful breathing exercises can help correct the chakras and promote a balanced flow of energy throughout the body and mind. Taking care of oneself regularly with physical, emotional, and spiritual components helps keep the seven primary chakras in balance and alignment.

Chapter 11

What Is Muladhara?

Chakras are energy centers in the body. However, most belief systems concur that seven main chakras run up your body along your spine. They start with the root chakra, which we'll discuss in detail in this chapter and book, and extend to the crown chakra, located at the crown of your head.

The concept of chakras originates from the idea that each person has two bodies in two parallel dimensions. The first one is the tangible body, which is located in the physical world. The second is the energy body, or subtle body, connected by energy pathways (or channels) known as nadi. These energy channels are connected and directed by nodes of psychic energy – or more commonly known as the chakras.

The physical body can affect the energy body (and vice versa), and this interaction is what allows you to balance your chakras.

Each of the seven major chakras has different physical and psychological effects on your body, meaning that any unbalanced chakra has a particular effect on your body. Learning what to look out for is the first step toward achieving a balanced body in both realms.

To start the balancing process, you should ideally start from the base one and carry on unblocking each chakra in order until you get to your crown chakra. So, to get you started, let's begin with understanding the root chakra.

What Is the Root Chakra?

As we've already told you, the Muladhara is found at the base of your spine. The word Muladhara —

the Sanskrit term– means root, hence its English name.

This chakra acts as the root of your body and is linked to the element of earth, which represents a person's ability to feel rooted and stable in life. It is connected to your familial relationships and sense of security. A healthy root chakra enables you to feel confident, safe, and secure as you go through the journey of life.

This chakra also supports your bone structure, acting as a connective chakra to the physical world around you. When the root chakra is blocked or unbalanced, all the other chakras in your body may go out of alignment.

The Root Chakra symbol.
In Hindu scripture and yogic texts, Muladhara is said to be the chakra from which the three main nadis (Ida, Pingala, Sushama) emerge. It is

considered to be the home of the god Ganpati - which is to say Ganpati governs it, and his influence on your life is considered to be spiritually emanating from the Muladhara. Along with being the god who brought good luck and removed obstacles, Ganpati is also the son of Shiva, who is described as the omniscient yogi who first taught yoga to Hindu sages.

The root chakra is where everything in your body begins. It is the home of your emotions. However, an unbalanced root chakra will lead to swings in your emotional state, including feelings of anger, insecurity, and restlessness. It can also cause your fear, panic, and anxiety levels to spike as a result of what your body sees as a threat to your safety and security.

An unbalanced root chakra is common for people who have had negative personal struggles, such as troubles with their financial situation, interpersonal relationships, and worries about ensuring their survival needs are met.

Another way the root chakra influences you is through its role in maintaining the constant flow of one's creativity. It acts as the root of creative intention in your body and, when in balance, ensures that a person feels confident to develop their ideas and inspiration. The root of your creativity is clear, allowing you to be able to bring your ideas to reality.

It allows you to stand up for yourself and your ideas and ensures you don't let the fear of failure hold you back. However, when unbalanced, it can make it challenging to bring your creative ideas to fruition, and there's a greater fear of defeat that can often stop you from trying in the first place.

Root Chakra and Sexuality

As mentioned above, your root chakra is located at the base of your spine – specifically, on your pelvic floor. This location also means that it significantly impacts your sexuality and sex life.

As we've discussed, one of the major effects of an out-of-balance root chakra is fear. When you're afraid, you're unable to open yourself up to intimacy, making it challenging to trust and connect with sexual partners. A blocked root chakra makes your sex life unsatisfying because you're unable to appreciate sex with a person you trust completely.

The root chakra also has physiological effects on your body. This is especially true for women who have experienced trauma in childhood. The root chakra responds by shutting down in women who are afraid of sex, whether it is because of previous traumas or worry about a painful first experience. A dormant root chakra also means the muscles in your pelvic floor tighten and can lead to a reduction in vaginal lubrication.

For women who have a sexual experience when their root chakra is closed, the tense pelvic floor muscles can cause pain and, in the case of first times, bleeding. This pain sets a precedent, causing you to expect it to reoccur the next time you have sex. This fear leads to an out-of-balance root chakra, which means both physiological and psychological reactions.

This combination of fear and physiological effects (tightened pelvic muscles) leads to long-term sexual dysfunction, which cannot be resolved until the root chakra is opened and balanced. For men, the fear and lack of trust in their partner leads to an unsatisfying sex life that, once again, requires their root chakra to be aligned and opened to remedy.

Understanding the Root Chakra in Depth

A red, four-petalled lotus with a yellow square in the center represents the Muladhara. Each petal has one of four Sanskrit letters (va, scha, sha, and sa) written in gold. Depending on the yogic tradition, these letters either symbolize the four vrittis (thoughts that surface in the mind) – natural pleasure, greatest joy, blissfulness in concentration, and delight in controlling passion – or represent dharma, artha, kama, and moksha.

At the center of the lotus, the syllable lam is placed within the yellow box. This is the bija mantra, or Vedic seed mantra, associated with the root chakra and will be discussed in further detail in other chapters in this book.

In some depictions of the root chakra symbol, eight spears point out from the sides and corners of the square towards the petals.

The root chakra is associated with the Hindu deity Ganpati, as discussed above, and the god Indra, who is the king of heaven and the god of the sky, weather, lightning, rains, and thunder.

As it is linked to the earth element, the root chakra is also associated with the color red (or pink), which symbolizes the earth. Additionally, it is linked to the sense of smell, and its musical note is C.

In your root chakras, you carry not only your own experiences but also ancestral memories, both good and bad. Thus, generational traumas can even affect people who have never experienced a similar level of hardship during their own lifetime, but balancing this chakra helps heal these deep-rooted traumas.

When energy flows unimpeded through your root chakra, the kundalini energy is awakened. The kundalini energy is the divine feminine energy associated with the goddess and lies dormant in the Muladhara until the chakra is opened. Energy flow through this chakra also gives the other six chakras a strong base they can lean on, which is why it's essential to start opening up your root chakra before any other.

Unbalanced Root Chakras

With an unbalanced root chakra, several physical and emotional problems can be prevalent in your lower body, including:

- Problems with the colon and bladder
- Constipation
- Pain in the pelvis
- Problems with your lower leg or feet
- Pain in the lower back
- Prostate problems in men
- Sleeping problems
- Weakened immunity, making it easier for you to fall ill
- Weight gain or weight loss

Psychological and emotional symptoms of an imbalanced root chakra include:

- Fear and loss of your sense of security
- Erratic behavior
- Negativity and cynicism

- Feeling extremely overwhelmed, like you're constantly living in survival mode
- Lack of energy and a constant feeling of lethargy
- Depression
- Anxiety disorders
- Eating disorders
- Lack of confidence and self-esteem
- Sudden inability to focus

You may also develop self-control issues, which is one of the reasons an unbalanced root chakra can lead to eating disorders – controlling your food intake can lead to a temporary feeling of regaining control but can actually lead to severe medical problems.

Furthermore, an imbalance may also lead to spiritual issues, such as an existential crisis or crisis of faith, loss of will, and a feeling of doubt about your place in the universe around you. It can lead to you losing interest in being part of the world.

A balanced root chakra, on the other hand, is linked to:

- The ability to connect with loved ones and feel grounded in your life
- Stability and security
- A healthy survival instinct
- A sense of belonging among the people around you

A healthy root chakra is essential for giving you the will to live and care for yourself and restore focus to your life. With a stable root chakra, you'll be able to thrive and truly meet your potential. Balancing your root chakra is key to regaining this sense of stability in your life. This book will explore ways to do so in detail in the following chapters, but some methods you can try include:

- Aromatherapy
- Crystal healing

- Yoga
- Meditation

You can also use movement, sound, and touch to balance your root chakra.

Movement is exactly what it sounds like – getting out of your home and moving around. As the root chakra is linked to the earth, it's recommended you engage with nature. Even something as simple as walking through a garden or hiking can help.

Another way to unblock your root chakra is by connecting to the ground with your feet. To do so, stand with a tennis ball on the ground in front of you. Then, shift one foot onto the ball, putting your weight on the other foot. Move the foot on the ball in a circular motion, allowing your ankle to move. When you feel grounded, change sides.

If spending time in nature isn't possible, other forms of movement, such as dance and pilates, can help as well.

You can also use sound to heal your chakras, including using singing bowls, sound baths, and gong sounds. As we'll cover later in the book, you can also use mantras. The root chakra's vibration frequency is 432 Hz; using sound at this vibration can help especially well.

Finally, you can also use touch to balance your chakra. This involves touching your body and being touched; one option is to try self-massage. Alternatively, you can ask a loved one for a massage or visit a professional. Being connected with another person by touch is a matter of trust, especially when being massaged. This helps you connect with other people better, allowing you to balance your root chakra.

You can also try other touch-based activities, including hugging (self-hugging is also an option), cuddling, and sex with a trusted partner. You should try touching your body through self-massages and self-hugs because this type of touch reinforces your love for yourself.

Besides self-touch, you should also set aside time to spend alone. You can work on your self-confidence and discover your true self. Use this time to manifest what you want from your life or spend it doing things that you enjoy but are otherwise unable to do due to a lack of time, such as reading a book, enjoying music, or going for a run. Essentially, you should do what helps whatever helps you to connect better with your inner, true, authentic self.

Why You Should Align Your Root Chakra

A balanced root chakra helps you feel more connected to the people around you and more secure in yourself and your place in the world.

However, there's more to it than just that.

An aligned, balanced root chakra ensures you feel a zest for life. It makes you enthusiastic about experiencing the world around you and rescues you from boredom and feelings of stagnation. It's also essential for you to feel energetic and able to complete your daily routine.

The root chakra also provides energy to the rest of the chakras in your body, so getting it balanced is critical for getting any of your chakras onto the same path.

Now that you understand your root chakra, it's time to look at it in further detail. The next chapter will explore the effects of a blocked root chakra and look at what can cause it.

It will also look at other issues with the root chakra, including the effects of a weak or overactive Muladhara. It will give you some symptoms to keep an eye out for and includes a questionnaire you can use to determine whether your root chakra is in balance.

Once you've worked out the state of your root chakra, you can then look at ways to address any imbalance that may exist. Other chapters will explore, in detail, some popular ways to treat imbalanced chakras and open closed Muladharas, including how to meditate, to open it, what mantras and affirmations you can use, and what mudras and pranayamas are recommended for your root chakra.

We also look at some yoga poses and sequences that can balance your Muladhara and list some crystals and stones you can incorporate into your meditation and yoga practice. Furthermore, you'll be able to learn how to use aromatherapy and essential oils to encourage the balancing process, and you'll be informed about which essential oils are best for this chakra.

One important thing this book will explore is how to tailor your diet to ensure your root chakra is balanced. Your diet and nutrition can have a significant impact on the state of your chakras, and this book will provide you will all the information you need to continue having a healthy diet while also taking care of your Muladhara.

By the time you're done with this book, you'll truly be a root chakra expert. You'll know how to balance your root chakra and be ready to move on to understanding the other chakras in your body.

So, what are you waiting for? Now that you know your root chakra, all that's left for you to do is turn the page and continue reading!

CHAPTER 12

Identify your Imbalance

Arya picked up her inquiry where she left off yesterday, asking it with the same excitement. You were telling me about the balances and imbalances of the chakras. The Sage, as usual, very calmly started to explain that to be able to balance your chakras, you can take two paths. The first requires you to identify the imbalances, identify which chakra is imbalanced and start balancing with that chakra. The second is where you directly start chakra balancing practices without thinking much about which one is imbalanced. Both approaches will ultimately lead to the alignment of all seven chakras. Arya, which one will you pick?

Arya thoughtfully answered, both sounds okay, but I would like to be more conscious of the changes in my life. And also, the sole purpose of meditation is to be more aware of oneself; therefore, I would choose the first approach. I will identify the imbalance first and then attune my energy accordingly.

Sage: Very well. I commend your decision to prioritize self-awareness and identifying imbalances. By taking this approach, you will be able to address any issues more effectively and bring about a deeper alignment of your chakras. Remember, self-reflection and mindfulness are key to this journey. Let's dive deeper into self-awareness.

Always know that there are three states of each chakra: balanced, blocked, and overactive. By understanding these states, you can better recognize when a chakra is imbalanced and take the necessary steps to bring it back into harmony. It's important to remember that each chakra influences different aspects of your physical, emotional, and spiritual well-being. By having your chakra blocked, you may experience physical ailments, emotional instability, and a lack of spiritual connection. On the other hand, an overactive chakra can lead to excessive energy in certain areas of your life, causing imbalance and potential burnout. Therefore, developing self-awareness and regularly assessing the state of your chakras are important.

Let's see the traits of all the chakras in all three states:

Root Chakra (Muladhar):

The root chakra is related to the basic sensation of safety. So, whenever you feel worried, afraid, insecure, or restless, you know this chakra is out of whack. You may also experience a loss of confidence in yourself. You begin to ignore yourself and your physical health, resulting in chronic pain and sickness. This may make you feel even more alienated, unconnected, and unsupported by others. As a result, if you don't keep an eye on it, it may exaggerate over time. Insecurity extends to financial insecurity; you struggle with money concerns, poverty mentality, or scarcity mentality. This chakra has a significant influence on your productivity.

And when this chakra is overactive, you have other problems, like becoming greedy, materialistic, or obsessed with comfort and security. You also tend to be more rigid, stubborn, or resistant to change. you experience aggression, anger, or become violent towards yourself or others too. Also, you may be overly attached to your possessions or identity. You may lust for power and control. All this in your nature pushes people around you away, leaving you less socially secure.

Also, you may experience physical symptoms like pain and stiffness in your lower back and hips.

So, whenever you experience any of the mentioned symptoms in your daily routines, please know that you need to work on your root chakra. And once you balance it, you will feel grounded and centered, and you will have a sense of stability within you. Also, you will have a healthier relationship with money and material resources. You will manage your money more efficiently. You will take care of your body and its needs. And you will have a sense of belonging and support from your family and community. Which will make you more safe and secure socially. Also, your productivity will improve significantly.

Sacral Chakra (Svadhisthan):

The primary feeling associated with this chakra is I feel. So, you would start to feel low all the time. You may lack the feel for life; you will not be able to focus. And would have overall negative thoughts and a negative outlook on life. This may be due to some trauma or life changing event from the past. Also, this chakra encapsulates creativity and ideas, so all the lack of ideas and inspiration you face is because this one is blocked. The fear of intimacy, difficulty forming relationships, low libido or lack of sexual desire, and guilt or shame around sexual pleasure indicate a blockage of this chakra. All the repressed and denied emotions pile up and further contribute to the blockage.

I'll give you a clue right now: you're a lady, and this chakra will undoubtedly be seriously out of balance. You'll feel a lot of unbalances just after giving birth, even at the most wonderful times. This chakra is highly impacted by the significant physical disruptions that your body experiences. Therefore, you will undoubtedly need to focus on your sacral chakra at some point in your life.

On the other hand, if this chakra is overactive, you will become overly emotional and experience frequent mood swings, which may attract drama and chaos in your life. You may have lowered your self-respect and started loosening up your boundaries. Also, you may develop sexual addiction or promiscuity. You will always search for pleasure, which may incline you towards drugs and addictive substances. You see, this is the reason why more people in the creative field are attracted to alcohol, cigarettes, and other addictive substances.

Endocrine difficulties, kidney and thyroid problems, lower back discomfort, anemia, PCOD, PMS, and general low energy levels are among the physical indications of sacral imbalance.

But when this chakra is in harmony, you feel blissful; you are enthusiastic and passionate. You're naturally good at coming up with ideas. Your libido and sexual arousal are both in good shape. You develop greater emotional intelligence, emotional stability, and interpersonal harmony. It makes it possible for you to enjoy life's joys and pleasures to the fullest.

Solar Plexus (Manipur):
This chakra is related to the basic sensation of I do. When it is blocked, your self-esteem plummets, you feel helpless over your life circumstances, and you develop an inferiority complex. You are unable to move on from the

past. Your self-assurance has entirely vanished. You also lack drive and a sense of direction in life, making it difficult to make decisions. You've been fatigued all day and lack the energy to do anything. Procrastination occurs regularly, and your productivity suffers as a result.

When this chakra is hyperactive, you become power hungry and develop dictatorial traits. You have a tendency to become a perfectionist and to be too critical of those around you. People think you're arrogant and egocentric, and your temper flares up regularly. You are primarily exhausted and anxious. The superhero Hulk is an example of an extremely active solar plexus.

Physically, you may be bothered by issues with your intestines and digestion.

And when this chakra is balanced, it helps you get through all of life's obstacles quite effortlessly. Your confidence and boldness shine through. You have a high sense of self-worth and self-esteem. Your life's goal and purpose become evident. You are capable of making decisions. You naturally become a leader and inspire others around you.

Arya interrupted, I have a quick question: You mentioned that the root chakra affects productivity and that a decline in productivity also denotes an imbalance in the solar plexus. How will I know which one to work on? The sage replies, I appreciate your attentiveness. Yes, productivity is associated with both the chakras I mentioned. When productivity suffers because you are constantly afraid of making mistakes, it indicates an imbalance in the root chakra. And when productivity suffers from a lack of energy and motivation to do anything, it is a sign of the solar plexus being imbalanced.

Arya: This requires one to be very aware of themselves. Sage: Yes, self-awareness is both the path and the goal. And don't worry; apart from explaining the traits of imbalances, I'll also give you a method to meditate and find your area or chakra to work on. First, let's complete the traits for the remaining chakras.

Heart Chaka (Anahat):

It should come as no surprise that the heart chakra focuses on our capacity for love and compassion, with I feel as its dominant sensation. You lack compassion and empathy if this chakra is blocked. You never have good things to say about people, and you have trouble building relationships. In general, you're feeling resentful and spiteful. You worry about being rejected and left behind. You start to remain irritable and unhappy in the face of excellent fortune. You also find it tough to forgive others and put your trust in them.

When this chakra becomes hyperactive, you become clingy, and your happiness becomes dependent on others. You are also overly helpful and self-sacrificing in your relationships, which leads to disappointment in the long run. You suffer from codependency, a loss of identity, and a lack of boundaries and self-care. You may also develop feelings of jealousy and possessiveness and begin to place unreasonable expectations on loved ones.
Breathing difficulties, nasal passage troubles, and heart diseases are examples of physical symptoms.

You become more serene, loving, and compassionate when this chakra is balanced. You begin to have relationships that are caring, harmonious, and meaningful. Acceptance and forgiveness of others, as well as forgiveness of yourself, come naturally to you. You value self-care and self-love. You also exude a more global sort of love for everyone and everything around you. You become more accepting of your environment.

Throat chakra (Vishudh):

This chakra is related to our capacity for vocal communication. The sense of I speak is at the center of everything. You may become withdrawn and quiet when blocked. Speaking your truth and expressing yourself may be challenging for you. You feel excluded and worry about being judged and misunderstood. You have a propensity to withdraw and might turn to deceit and lying. Your overall communication ability is inhibited.

But keep in mind that an introvert is someone who doesn't feel comfortable sharing their energies with others; never mistake this for having a clogged throat chakra. They may be excellent communicators, but they only choose to speak to certain people.

In an overactive state, you become loud and talkative. You unconsciously interrupt others and try to dominate conversations. You begin to use unpleasant, crude, blunt, and harsh language. You struggle with listening to people and being present. You may also turn to gossiping and spreading rumors. You also begin to argue and cuss a lot.

Physical symptoms include problems with the thyroid, mouth ulcers, and tonsils.

When this chakra is balanced, you become an excellent orator. People love to talk to you because you make them feel heard and still make others understand your point. You become expressive, honest, and a good communicator. Integrity and truthfulness come naturally to you. You are also more respectful toward everyone around you.

Third Eye Chakra (Ajna):

Your intuition, insight, and the overarching sense of I see are all governed by this chakra. Confusion and a lack of clarity may occur when this chakra is obstructed. You can have a very short attention span and be constantly distracted and indecisive. You might start to see most things with skepticism and close-mindedness. and could have poor short- and long-term vision.

When this chakra is overactive, you could have delusions and paranoia. Additionally, you have nightmares and hallucinations. Additionally, it can be challenging to distinguish between truth and fiction. You can develop a fascination with psychic phenomena.

You could experience migraines and headaches as bodily symptoms. Additionally, you can get sinus or eye issues or tumors in the brain.

Being in balance with this chakra makes you more perceptive, smart, and intuitive. You learn to focus on the big picture without losing sight of the minutiae. You also have a distinct life vision and purpose. Like a youngster, you approach everything with curiosity and an open mind.

Crown chakra (Sahasrar):
This chakra governs the connection to the divine and higher realms. The primary emotion is I understand. When this chakra is blocked, you feel cut off from spirituality and a higher power. You perceive life as useless and lacking in inspiration. You believe in cynicism and nihilism, which means you perceive everything as self-serving and lacking in religion and values.

When this chakra is overactive, you have a sense of disconnection from reality or the physical world. You are subjected to dogmatism and extremism. You may acquire an addiction to spiritual activities and narcotics, causing you to rely solely on God and do nothing. You develop arrogance and a sense of superiority as well.

Nerve pain, hair loss, memory loss, Alzheimer's, cognitive function issues, or epilepsy are some of the physical signs. You may also feel estranged from your higher self, purpose or the divine.

Enlightenment, spirituality, and conscious feelings may be experienced when this chakra is balanced. A connection to the divine and higher worlds increases awareness and knowledge of oneself and others. Life's bliss and happiness are unity and harmony with all that is.

These were all the characteristics for each chakra to identify your imbalance, then. Sage added, Let me tell you one more thing: if these imbalanced characteristics continue for a long time, they may start to affect other chakras and make them imbalanced too. So start addressing any imbalances as soon as you even remotely identify with them.

Arya: How can I recognize them when they simply appear? The characteristics may not be apparent, or I might not be in the right frame of mind to perceive them. Sage: Yes, you may sometimes be in a state of denial, which is very typical when you have imbalances. Additionally, when the chakras first begin to go out of balance, the features may not be as obvious. Consider the imbalance as a scale of numbers. It is blocked on the extreme left, balanced in the center, and hyperactive on the extreme right. And on the scale, your imbalance might be somewhere in between. Let's really begin recognizing them and addressing them with the use of a brief meditation. Follow my instructions with full faith.

CHAPTER 13

Finding your imbalance via meditation

Sage: Arya, to begin this practice, let's close our eyes and take a few deep breaths. Inhale slowly and exhale gently, allowing your body to relax with each breath. Arya followed the sage's instructions, her breath becoming a soothing rhythm that carried her into a state of deep relaxation. As she breathed, she felt the tension in her body melt away, leaving her calm and centered.

Sage, with a soft tone, started to guide her. Now, I want you to imagine a warm, radiant light surrounding you, cocooning you in a comforting embrace. Feel the energy of this light, like a gentle hug from the universe itself. Arya's imagination took flight, and she envisioned herself bathed in a soothing golden light. She felt safe and embraced by the universe's love.

Sage, with this warm light surrounding you, let's journey within. Slowly turn your attention to the base of your spine. This is the location of your root chakra, Muladhara. Imagine a vibrant red energy swirling in this area. As you focus on it, notice any sensations or feelings that arise. Is there any stiffness or tension in this part of your body?

Arya turned her awareness to the base of her spine, picturing the swirling red energy. She took note of the sensations in that area. The sage watched her with a kind smile, allowing her time to explore.

Sage, Good, Arya. Now, let's move our attention to the area just below your navel. This is your sacral chakra, Svadhishthana. Imagine bright orange energy swirling here. Observe any sensations or tension in this region.

Arya shifted her focus to the area below her navel, imagining the vibrant orange energy. She sensed a subtle tightness there and made a mental note. Sage very gently appreciated her. You're doing well, Arya. Now, let's ascend to your stomach area, your solar plexus chakra, Manipura. Imagine brilliant yellow energy spinning here. Pay attention to any sensations that arise.

Arya turned her awareness to her stomach, visualizing the yellow energy swirling. She noticed a bit of tension in her stomach and acknowledged it without judgment. Sage, moving upward, we arrive at your heart center, Anahata. Imagine soothing green energy filling this space. Feel its gentle vibrations and become aware of any sensations in your heart area.

Arya focused on her heart, visualizing the calming green energy. She felt a warmth spreading through her chest, and a smile graced her lips. Sage said softly, You're progressing beautifully, Arya. Now, let's ascend to your throat, your throat chakra, Vishuddha. Picture a serene blue energy swirling here. Notice any sensations or tightness in your throat region.

Arya's attention shifted to her throat, where she pictured the serene blue energy. She became aware of a subtle constriction in her throat and acknowledged it with curiosity. Sage, Well done, Arya. Now, let's journey to your forehead and your third-eye chakra, Ajna. Imagine indigo energy spinning here. Take note of any sensations or feelings in this area.

Arya directed her focus to her forehead, visualizing the indigo energy swirling. She sensed a gentle pressure between her eyebrows, a sensation she had never noticed before. Sage encourages her: You're gaining insight into your own energy centers. Finally, let's ascend to the crown of your head, your crown chakra, Sahasrara. Imagine divine violet energy radiating here. Feel its connection to the universe and any sensations you experience.

Arya turned her awareness to the crown of her head, picturing the divine violet energy. She felt a gentle tingling sensation at the top of her head, as if she were connecting to something greater than herself. Sage gently smiled and said, Arya, you've completed the journey through your chakras. Take a few deep breaths and slowly bring your awareness back to the present moment.

Arya followed the sage's guidance, taking deep breaths and allowing herself to transition back to the serene forest setting. As she opened her eyes, she felt a sense of clarity and connection she had never experienced before.

Sage: Arya, you've embarked on a journey of self-discovery and self-awareness. By noticing the sensations and tension in each chakra, you gain insight into areas that might need a little extra attention and care. With practice and mindfulness, you can work towards balancing and harmonizing these energy centers, contributing to your overall well-being.

Arya smiled, her heart filled with gratitude for the wisdom the sage had shared. As they sat by the bubbling brook, surrounded by the beauty of nature, Arya felt a deeper connection to herself and the universe, ready to continue her journey of growth and understanding.

Arya followed the sage's guidance, taking deep breaths and allowing herself to transition back to the serene forest setting. As she opened her eyes, she felt a sense of clarity and connection she had never experienced before.

Sage: Arya, you've embarked on a journey of self-discovery and self-awareness. By noticing the sensations and tension in each chakra, you gain insight into areas that might need a little extra attention and care. With practice and mindfulness, you can work towards balancing and harmonizing these energy centers, contributing to your overall well-being.

Arya curiously asked I've noticed that you associated specific colors with each chakra during our meditation. Why did you choose those particular colors? Sage smiled and replied. Ah, an excellent question, Arya. The colors associated with each chakra hold deeper significance and symbolism. They help us connect with the energy and qualities that each chakra represents.

Sage continued that not only colors but each chakra has several different things like seed sounds, frequencies, symbols, primary feelings, etc. associated with it. Through which we work on each chakra. As usual, I'll tell you the importance of each associated thing if you are consistent and come tomorrow.

Chapter 14

Throat Chakra - Communication

Chapter Five deals with the throat chakra, which will highlight the aspect of communication throughout the chapter. This communication is specifically directed at your higher self, how you can tap into this realm of your being, and how to notice when the throat chakra is not in alignment.

The Importance of Communication

Communication is the most important tool to making your feelings known, but what happens when there is no one to discuss these feelings with, or you fail to openly express these feelings? Do you simply disregard these feelings and pretend they do not exist, or do you seek other ways to get them across to someone who might care to listen? Using the throat chakra to communicate what needs to be said requires that you first learn how to speak to yourself. Not only by overloading your mind with all the thoughts that are already running in it but by also observing anything inside of you that may arise from this communication.

The throat chakra is the center of your communication, which is also known as *Vishuddha* (purest). It is associated with the ether, where purification and expression are the roots of this chakra. Blue is the color that represents the throat chakra, so you might wish to drape yourself in blue clothing, spend time watching the sky or sea, or simply imagine all the things that bring you to a state of peace when you wish to bring this chakra to alignment.

A balanced throat chakra enables you to meditate with ease, where the energy you create from within gets used effectively. The importance of communication is noticeable in the relief you get from speaking your mind; the more open someone may become from you expressing yourself or how carefully you choose and use your words. Even when you are establishing a connection with yourself, communication is still vital. It encourages you to ask questions about yourself that only you can explore honest answers to, and you might just be surprised by the answers you find. The essence of positive self-talk is to also make your inner voice more audible for you to hear it when it is needed. This inner voice is linked to your higher self, so you would need to find this voice to fully experience your higher self.

Connecting With Your Higher Self

Your higher self is what makes up your mind, body, spirit, and heart, where all of these are interconnected for the enhancement of the essence of your true self. There is no point in your body or picture of yourself where you can highlight your higher self, as this is a holistic experience of your being. This holistic experience is channeled through the activation of your chakras, specifically where your throat chakra is awakened once you speak your truth.

The use of the chant 'Ham' (pronounced as 'Hum') can help activate the throat chakra, or you may choose to express yourself by using the words 'I speak…' to bring things to action through the power of your words. You might also wish to use the 741 Hz energy frequency for aligning this chakra since it encourages the awakening of your intuition. The vibrations from the insect-like sounds and rhythm of the 741 Hz solfeggio frequency may transfer these vibrations to and through your entire being as well. Your diet might be influenced to change, as this frequency emphasizes living a simple and healthy life, along with bringing purity and stability to your spiritual life.

A great way to reflect on the communications you have with yourself is by writing down your words as a form of self-talk. Journaling is one of the tools that are most effective for communicating since you would be relaying your thoughts and feelings into words that you can later read to make sense of once you have released them. This interaction with yourself will enable you to also tap into your mind and develop a better understanding of it. This reflection exercise will also help you to be openly honest with yourself. When you reach a milestone in communicating with yourself, you will equally influence your communication with others. You will also see what areas of your life need transformation and which have become more enhanced during this process.

You can also find a quiet spot to sit down and close your eyes for a few minutes, where you try to picture yourself in your happiest state. Do you know what made you this happy or why this is a pleasant feeling for you? Ask yourself if you have ever experienced this feeling before and notice how it makes you feel in the present moment.

Try to notice significant features in the environment you are in by considering:

- If you are alone or with a specific other
- If you are doing any activity and what it is
- The sounds that surround you
- Then monitor your state of being in your vision and reality

Speaking up about anything bothering you is also a good way to clear the throat chakra energy. Being vocal about your truth instead of allowing other people to have the power of silencing you will encourage you to find your voice in the world. This may encourage the development of your confidence and improved self-esteem too.

Having a positive outlook on yourself, your life, and the world around you should not in any way be viewed as an attempt to block out the negativity of the world. Instead, a positive outlook should be viewed as a way to carve out the way you wish things to be. This is why it all begins in the mind—with you. When considering your emotional intelligence, for example, you may find that it is hard for you to deal with certain emotions not because of the ease that comes with running away from them, but the inability to start addressing these emotions as they arise may be from your general unawareness of them. When you become aware of your emotional well-being, you can find it a lot easier to tend to your mental, social, spiritual, and physical well-being as well. This is possible because interlinking effects are associated with each aspect that our being comprises.

So, while you may think that harboring your feelings and emotions is protecting yourself from making these become known, you may unconsciously be causing your heart chakra and throat chakra to become imbalanced. This may also cause other people to sense this about you and find it easy to take advantage of you because of how accepting you are or quiet about situations that do not necessarily sit well with you. No part of your life experience should ever be reduced to you cutting off your words to accommodate the feelings of the next person, especially if their words or actions might have been the cause of your consideration of remaining mum when you are feeling unsettled. Instead, create a habit of having positive self-talk with yourself, which will instinctively become the positive talk you have with other people. Positive self-talk will also help you feel good about yourself and value your worth and the impact you make by being alive. The mind will begin to register how beneficial this self-talk is to your well-being. It will also create a repetitive pattern of reminding you not to forget or disregard this. The only way you can share positivity in a world infested with negativity is to be that voice for positivity—so choose to be the one thing that is good about your life or your day. It is also quite a good health tip to ensure that you feel good before making others feel good.

Singing and humming are some of the best ways to clear the throat chakra. Whether you have an angelic singing voice or you can hardly hold a note, singing is helpful for everyone who tries it out. When you sing or hum, the vibrations sent throughout your whole body awaken senses inside you that release happy hormones. The frequency of the song may help with awakening other chakras as well, and this could help you bring a balance to more than just the throat chakra. If possible, try to hit those notes as high as you possibly can, as this will alert every part of your body to come alive. You could also sense a frequency change or ringing in your ears from the 'shock' that your body might experience from the sudden noise of your voice, and this is entirely okay. This will simply mean that you would be doing something out of the ordinary that your energy now has to adjust to, based on whether it is beneficial for it or not.

You can also stretch out your neck in a slow up and down motion of your head to flex the throat chakra. You should try not to lean your head backward too much, as this may cause you

www.ingramcontent.com/pod-product-compliance
Lightning Source LLC
LaVergne TN
LVHW010220070526
838199LV00062B/4674